Revitalize Your Life

Immune-boosting Fitness and Nutrition Habits

Table of Contents

Chapter 1. Introduction

In this empowering Special Report titled "Revitalize Your Life: Immune-boosting Fitness and Nutrition Habits," we chart the journey towards a more vibrant and healthful existence! With an engaging blend of practical strategies and science-backed insights, our report is designed to make fitness and nutrition not just more accessible but also pleasurable. It offers a roadmap for those yearning to tap into the magic of daily nutritional habits and targeted fitness exercises that can enhance immunity and promote boundless health. Crafted by top health experts and coaches, this life-changing guide is a treasure trove of information laying out all the delicious meals, vital nutrient sources, and fun exercises that can propel you from languid to lively. Get ready to revolutionize the way you look at health—turn the first page and take your first step towards reenergizing your life!

Chapter 2. Unlocking the Power of Nutrition: Superfoods for Immunity

Understanding the immune-boosting potential of superfoods is paramount to revitalizing and nurturing your health. Fueling your body with nutritious foods packed with vitamins, minerals, and antioxidants can create a line of defense protecting you from illness, fortifying your overall wellbeing, and fostering vibrant energy. Below, we detail superfoods that uplift your immune health and provide helpful tips weaved into the culinary landscape.

2.1. The Power of Antioxidants

Many superfoods are rich in antioxidants that protect your cells from damage and promote optimal body functioning. Berries such as blueberries, strawberries, and acai berries contain high levels of antioxidants. Include them in your breakfast routine or whip them into a nourishing smoothie for a tasty immune-boosting treat!

Citrus fruits, loaded with vitamin C, also make powerful antioxidants. Our bodies cannot produce or store vitamin C, so it's vital to include generous amounts of citrus fruits like oranges, limes, grapefruits, and lemons in our daily diet.

2.2. Harnessing the Might of Minerals

Zinc and selenium are important minerals that boost your immune system. Beautifully enough, nature provides us with superfoods that house these microelements.

Oysters are champions in the zinc league, but for the more everyday meal, lean meat, poultry, seafood, milk, whole grain products, beans, seeds, and nuts are excellent sources. For selenium, rely on brazil nuts, fish such as halibut and sardines, and enriched whole grains.

2.3. Beta Carotene: The Colorful Defender

Beta carotene is another important antioxidant that supports immune health. Converted into vitamin A in our bodies, it helps fortify the immune system against infections. Orange-colored fruits and vegetables, like sweet potatoes, carrots, bell peppers, and cantaloupes, are packed with beta carotene. Leafy greens such as spinach and kale are also good sources.

2.4. Lean on Legumes and Nuts

Beans, lentils, and chickpeas are not only brimful of protein—essential for repairing body cells—but also contain other immune-boosting nutrients like fiber, magnesium and iron. Nuts, particularly almonds, have a high concentration of Vitamin E, a potent antioxidant.

2.5. The Importance of a Balanced Diet

While these superfoods can enhance your immunity, they aren't miracle potions in and of themselves. Maintaining a balanced diet that supports all body functions is crucial for optimal health. Embrace a diverse palette of fruits, vegetables, lean meats, whole grains, and legumes to ensure you absorb a full spectrum of nutrients.

2.6. Cooking Techniques for Maximum Nutrition Retention

Eating nutritious food isn't enough; you also need to cook it properly to retain its nutritional value. For instance, avoid overcooking vegetables, as it can lead to vitamin loss. Many nutrients are water-soluble, so boiling might result in loss of vitamins into the cooking water. Opt for steaming, grilling, or roasting instead.

2.7. Proactive Dietary Changes: A Stepping Stone to Better Health

Changing your dietary habits may seem challenging initially. Start with small, manageable steps, such as incorporating one extra serving of fruits or vegetables into your meal each day. Gradually make healthier substitutions, like swapping refined grains with whole grains.

2.8. Hydration: An Unsung Hero

Water plays a crucial role in facilitating essential bodily functions, including digestion and nutrient absorption, making it a vital contributor to your immunity. Aim to drink at least 8 glasses of water daily.

Each stride you take towards an improved diet replenishes your immune system and equips you with vigor for life's adventures. Remember, nourishing your body is a form of self-respect, and as you glow in robust health, you'll find the energy to embrace life to its fullest!

Chapter 3. Morning Regimes: Kickstart Your Day with Energizing Routines

Just as a well-tuned vehicle creates a robust and comfortable ride, a fine-tuned body fuels us with unparalleled vitality. Starting your day strong means creating a morning routine centred around energizing exercises and nutritious meals. This chapter helps you design habits that awaken your inner resilience and invigorate your body and mind for the day ahead.

3.1. The Power of A Morning Exercise Routine

The first light of day can be an ideal time for exercising. The advantages of morning workouts go beyond the obvious benefit of freeing time for other activities later. They act as an internal wake-up call, laying a firm foundation of energy for the day.

If you're new to exercise or have specific health considerations, seek advice from a healthcare provider before starting an exercise regimen. Here are some recommendations:

Daily Stretching: Take the first 5-10 minutes of your day to engage in full-body stretching. This practice increases muscular flexibility, stimulates circulation and promotes a sense of calm. Head-to-toe stretches or yoga sequences, particularly sun salutations, are ideal for starters.

Cardiovascular Exercises: Cardio has proven benefits for heart health. Try 25-30 minutes of brisk walking, jogging, cycling, or skipping to pump your metabolism and heart rate. While rigorous for some, these exercises can be modified according to one's physical capacity.

Circuit training: A combination of strength and cardio exercises that can be adjusted for any fitness level. Consider working out with bodyweight exercises such as burpees, push-ups, or lunges, alternating these with short bouts of high-intensity cardio.

3.2. Breakfast: Breaking the Fast Right

An energy-rich morning meal sets the right tone for the day and replenishes your body's glucose supply after the night's fast. It also helps maintain concentration, mood, and physical stamina throughout the day. Here are some power-packed breakfast options:

Overnight oats with chia seeds and berries: This nutrient-dense meal includes complex carbohydrates, antioxidants, fiber, omega-3 fats, and high-quality protein.

Egg scramble with spinach and avocado: Offering a well-rounded mix of proteins, vitamins, and healthy fats, this dish aids in building muscle, strengthening immunity, and promoting heart health.

Smoothie bowls: A colorful blend of fruits, seeds, and yogurt, these are not only tasty but also packed with vitamins, antioxidants, and probiotics for gut health.

3.3. Hydration: Don't Miss Out on Your Morning Elixir

Staying hydrated is paramount for maintaining bodily functions, boosting metabolism, and promoting skin health. Start your day with a glass of water; it activates internal organs, helps flush out toxins, and primes your system for the day.

Infusing water with lemon, cucumber, or mint adds nutritional benefits while delivering a refreshing morning taste. Additionally, green tea and herbal infusions are excellent sources of antioxidants and a superb substitute if plain water seems monotonous.

3.4. Mindfulness Practice: Clear Your Head for the Day

In addition to physical exercise and nutrition, mental wellness is an integral part of health. It's remarkable how much power a simple practice of mindfulness can have over our physical and mental health.

Meditation: Practicing 10-15 minutes of meditation in the morning can drastically reduce stress levels and promote clarity and focus.

Gratitude journaling: Start your day by jotting down a few things you're grateful for: it sets a positive tone, encourages an optimistic mentality, and reduces stress.

Deep breathing: Deep, slow, controlled breathing exercises are effective in calming the mind, reducing anxiety, and promoting focus and awareness.

This ends the first chapter of your progressive journey towards a revitalized life. Incorporating these energizing morning routines into your daily life can significantly transform your health, boosting both physical and mental strength. Remember, consistency is key - strive to commit to these habits daily. You are on the way to a more vibrant, healthful existence - a brighter morning is just the start!

Chapter 4. Exercise Your Way to Better Immunity: A Deep Dive

Exercise may sometimes be the last thing on your mind when you're feeling under the weather. However, regular, moderate-intensity exercise is beneficial for your immune system. It can fend off infections and diseases, as well as help you heal faster if you do get sick.

4.1. Understanding the Immune System

Our immune system is a sophisticated defense system that helps us fight off infections. It consists of two interactive parts: the innate immune system, which is our first line of defense against pathogens, and the adaptive immune system, which develops a targeted response to specific threats. Regular exercise can help both parts work more effectively.

Various cells are involved in the immune response. These include white blood cells, such as lymphocytes, which can recognize and destroy particular antigens, and phagocytes, which engulf infectious agents. Moderate exercise can cause these cells to circulate more rapidly, which means they may be able to detect and fight pathogens sooner.

4.2. The Scientific Connection Between Exercise and Immunity

Exercising regularly has been linked to a range of long-term health benefits, including a healthier immune system. Exercise has a unique ability to boost the immune system by enhancing immune regulation and reducing inflammation.

Several studies have discovered that moderate-intensity physical activities, such as walking, bicycling, or swimming, can increase the circulation of important immune cells in your body, like natural killer cells and T cells. This helps your body find and defeat potential pathogens and cancer cells faster.

Additionally, continuous exercise can delay the onset of immunosenescence, which is a slow, gradual decrease in immune function that comes with age. Maintaining a regular physical activity regimen can keep your immune system running smoothly well into your golden years.

4.3. Best Exercises for Boosting Immunity

The best kind of exercise for immune health is moderate in intensity and regular in frequency.

1. **Aerobic exercises**: Activities like jogging, swimming, and cycling are great for your cardiovascular health as well as your immune system. These exercises increase the circulation of immune cells enabling them to perform their tasks efficiently.

2. **Resistance training**: This type of exercise strains your muscles, forcing them to repair and grow stronger. During the repair process, your body releases several different types of cells and molecules that support your immune system.

3. **Flexibility exercises**: Activities like yoga and stretching help keep your body agile and reduce the risk of injury. Additionally, these practices often emphasize breathing and mindfulness, which can help reduce stress—a known immune suppressor.

Remember, consistency is key. Aim for at least 150 minutes of moderate-intensity exercise or 75 minutes of vigorous-intensity exercise a week.

4.4. The Impact of Overtraining on Immune System

While regular exercise is beneficial, pushing too hard can have the opposite effect. Intense, prolonged training without proper recovery can suppress your immune function and leave you more prone to infections.

Acute bouts of extreme exercise, especially without adequate rest and diet, can lead to a temporary decline in immune function, known as "open window" phenomenon. This can last anywhere from 3 to 72 hours post-exercise and increase the likelihood of developing an infection during this recovery phase.

So, how do you avoid overtraining? Monitor your body's reaction to your training load. If you notice signs of overreaching like a persistent heavy, tired feeling in your muscles or a drop in performance, add more recovery days to your routine.

4.5. Eating to Support Your Immune System and Exercise

A healthy diet complements a good exercise routine. Complete, balanced nutrition is necessary to support your immune system during and after exercise.

Incorporate plenty of fruits and vegetables in your diet. They are packed with vitamins, minerals, and antioxidants, which protect your immune cells from damage. Rich sources of vitamin C, like citrus fruits and bell peppers, can especially bolster your immunity.

Don't forget about protein. This nutrient is crucial for recovery and repair after workouts, and some proteins (like casein and whey) can also support immune function.

Always hydrate well, especially during and after workouts, to replace fluids lost through sweating.

4.6. In Conclusion

Regular, moderate-intensity exercise is powerful medicine for your immune system. It can strengthen your immunity, helping you recover from illnesses faster or avoid them altogether. But remember, balance is key—overtraining can suppress your immunity. So listen to your body, allow yourself plenty of time to rest and recover, and fuel your body with nutrient-dense foods to support both your immune system and your physical goals.

With consistency and balance, exercise can be an enjoyable, natural, and effective way to bolster your immunity and revitalize your life. What are you waiting for? Lace up your shoes and get moving!

Chapter 5. Hydration and Health: The Life-Sustaining Duo

When it comes to maintaining health and boosting our immune system, it is easy to overlook the seemingly simple act of staying properly hydrated. However, hydration plays a vital role in the functioning of every system in our body—from warming us up when we are cold, to cooling us down when we are hot, from ensuring our heart functions efficiently, to enabling cellular regeneration and growth.

5.1. The Importance of Hydration

Water is not called the essence of life without reason. Our bodies are composed of about 60% water, and this vital substance is involved in nearly every bodily function. Hydrating has major implications for our general health, which includes strengthening the immune system, aiding digestion, maintaining brain function, and improving physical performance.

Consider it as the transportation system of the body. It delivers nutrients, bolts of energy, and even commands from the brain to the rest of the body. It escorts out waste materials and toxins which, if accumulated, can dampen our immune response and make our bodies a breeding ground for diseases and infections.

If we look at the engine of this intricate transportation system, known as metabolism, we'll find that it requires adequate hydration as well. Water is essential in the function of mitochondria, the powerhouse of our cells, where food is converted into energy. Dehydration can slow down this process and lead to feelings of lethargy and fatigue.

5.2. Understanding Dehydration

Dehydration occurs when the body loses more fluids than it intakes. This imbalance disrupts normal body functions and if severe, can be life-threatening. Dehydration doesn't just occur from lack of drinking water. It can also happen as a result of excessive sweating, diarrhea, vomiting, diabetes, and frequent urination.

Common signs of dehydration include thirst, less frequent urination, dark-colored urine, fatigue, dizziness, and confusion. Chronic dehydration can lead to complications like urinary tract infections, kidney stones, and even kidney failure.

5.3. How Much Water Do We Need?

A common recommendation is to drink eight 8-ounce glasses of water a day, which equals about 2 liters, or half a gallon, often referred to as the 8×8 rule. However, individual needs can vary greatly based on factors such as age, sex, weight, physical activity, and overall health.

For instance, if you're physically active, pregnant, breastfeeding, or ill, your hydration requirements may be higher. Use urine color as a general guide to assess your hydration status. Pale, straw-colored urine indicates adequate hydration, while darker colored urine might mean you need to drink more water.

5.4. Hydrating Beyond Plain Water

While water is, of course, a primary source of hydration, it's not the only one. Many foods and other beverages also contribute to your daily water intake. Fruits and vegetables with high water content, herbal teas, and even soups support hydration. It is also pivotal to remember that certain drinks like caffeinated beverages and alcohol can cause more frequent urination, and hence, might augment the risk of dehydration.

5.5. Exercise and Hydration

Exercise sparks the production of sweat as the body's cooling mechanism which, in turn, results in the loss of body water. Furthermore, intensive exercise can also lead to electrolyte imbalance due to excess sweating. Staying hydrated before, during, and after exercise is crucial to maintaining performance and avoiding heat-related illnesses.

5.6. Hydration for a Robust Immune System

A well-hydrated system allows the body to transport immune-boosting nutrients and hormones to cells easier, eliminating waste products and defending cells against harmful pathogens. Water also aids the production of lymph, a fluid that forms part of the immune system helping to circulate white blood cells and nutrients to the body tissues.

5.7. Conclusion

In concluding, it becomes clear that hydration stands as a central pillar in our overall health and well-being. Proper hydration helps our bodies function at their highest potential, and consequently, bear the flag of our immunity high and strong under varying conditions. Remember, every sip of water contributes to a healthier, more vibrant life! So, take that glass of water and make a toast to your health.

Chapter 6. Sleep Tight, Boost Right: The Impact of Rest on Immunity

Sound, sufficient sleep is crucial to maintaining optimal health, and its far-reaching effects on our immune system cannot be overstated. Our body's defenses burn the midnight oil, working diligently while we peacefully slumber, ensuring that we wake up re-energized and ready to tackle the upcoming day.

6.1. Understanding Sleep

Sleep is not a passive activity. Far from it, when we fall asleep, our bodies launch into a series of complex processes. Neurotransmitters and hormones are released, initiating various phases of sleep that are imperative for us to feel rested. Simultaneously, the human body repairs tissues, develops muscle, and restores energy. Needless to say, our immune system is a key participant in this nocturnal orchestra.

6.2. The Sleep-Immunity Connection

Research has constantly highlighted the deep-rooted relationship between sufficient sleep and a robust immune system. During sleep, the immune system releases proteins called cytokines. Certain cytokines protect against inflammation and infection, thus playing a crucial role in immune response. Lack of adequate sleep diminishes cytokine production, leaving us susceptible to illness. Furthermore, infection-fighting antibodies and cells decrease when we are sleep-deprived. It's clear that compromised sleep can lead to a weakened immune response, making us more vulnerable to viruses and bacteria.

6.3. The Detriments of Sleep Deprivation

Sleep deprivation has become a rampant issue in today's hustle culture. It does more than just leave you feeling groggy and grumpy. Chronic sleep deficiency is linked with various health issues, including heart disease, diabetes, obesity, and a weakened immune system. It hampers your body's ability to respond promptly to immune challenges and makes recovery from illness slower. It's essential to understand the detrimental effects of missing out on rest to comprehend fully why prioritizing sleep is as vital as maintaining a healthy diet and regular exercise.

6.4. Quality of Sleep

While the duration of sleep is fundamental, the quality should not be overlooked either. Quality sleep involves spending appropriate durations in all sleep stages, especially deep sleep and REM sleep, both of which play imperative roles in promoting health and boosting immunity. Numerous factors can affect your sleep quality, including your sleep environment, dietary habits, and lifestyles such as screen usage before bedtime. These factors can cause sleep disruptions that deprive your body of the chance to rejuvenate fully.

6.5. Sleep Hygiene: The Road to Better Sleep

Improving sleep hygiene can significantly enhance both sleep quantity and quality. This includes maintaining a consistent sleeping schedule, even on weekends and holidays; ensuring a dark, quiet, and cool environment for sleeping; restricting screen time prior to sleep; indulging in a relaxing pre-sleep routine; and avoiding large meals, caffeine, and alcohol before bedtime.

6.6. Exercise and Sleep

Regular exercise can work wonders for sleep. Besides tiring you out, enabling you to fall asleep faster, it also promotes prolonged deep sleep, the restorative stage of sleep. Thus, regular physical activity benefits not just your overall health but also your sleep and, consequently, your immunity.

6.7. Nutrition for Good Sleep

Your dietary habits significantly impact your sleep quality. Certain foods and drinks contain components that can interfere with sleep. Conversely, there are nutrients, notably tryptophan, magnesium, and calcium that aid in sleep by contributing to the production of melatonin, the sleep hormone.

6.8. The Role of Stress

Stress is a significant sleep disruptor. It triggers the release of cortisol, a hormone that interferes with sleep. Finding effective ways to manage stress, such as meditation, yoga, mindfulness, deep breathing, or even keeping a gratitude journal, can help foster better sleep.

6.9. The Magic of Napping

While it may not replace quality night-time sleep, napping can provide a considerable boost to your immune system. A study found that a thirty-minute nap could reverse the hormonal impact of a night of poor sleep.

We cannot overemphasize the importance of sleep for immunity. It's high time we recognize sleep as a formidable ally to our immune defenses. By implementing good sleep hygiene and mindful habits, we can ensure that we are giving our bodies the rest they require to keep us healthy, vibrant, and ready to face life's challenges. Remember, when it comes to boosting immunity, every good day begins with a good night's sleep.

Chapter 7. Meal Planning for Immunity: Designing Your Personal Wellness Menu

Before we delve into the specifics of planning meals for immunity, let's shed light on the concept of immunity. The immune system is the body's defensive network designed to keep you safe from harmful pathogens such as viruses and bacteria. Certain food items, effective dietary practices, and lifestyle changes can bolster it. A diet rich in fruits, vegetables, lean proteins, and whole grains can provide vital nutrients, thereby boosting your immune system.

7.1. Understanding the Immune-Boosting Nutrients

A number of beneficial nutrients play critical roles in supporting your immune system. Let's unpack these nutrition heroes:

Vitamins: Key vitamins essential for maintaining robust immunity include Vitamin A, C, D, and E. Vitamins A and D are fat soluble and mainly work within cells to strengthen the body's response to infections. Vitamin C, a cornerstone of immune health, boosts the formation of antibodies that bind to foreign invaders in the body while Vitamin E, a powerful antioxidant, protects your cells from oxidative damage.

Minerals: Selenium, zinc, iron, and copper are all vital minerals for immunity. They not only aid in the growth and repair of bodily tissues, but also assist in wound healing and infection prevention.

Probiotics: These beneficial bacteria aid digestion and help maintain gut health, which is critical for immune function as the intestinal tract houses approximately 70% of all immune cells within the body.

Foods rich in these immune-boosting nutrients should become pillars of your wellness menu.

7.2. Designing Your Personal Wellness Menu

Now that you're aware of the nutrients needed for immune health, it's time you learn how to incorporate them into your meal planning.

Pre-Breakfast – Kickstart your Day: Begin your day with a glass of warm lemon water. Lemons are rich in Vitamin C, which aids in fighting off infections.

Breakfast – Fuel Up: A smoothie bowl jam-packed with fruits like berries, kiwi, and banana, topped with a sprinkle of seeds, offers you a nutrient-dense start. This meal is high in Vitamins A, C, and E, plus iron and zinc.

Lunch – Balance and Satisfy: Lunch could comprise grilled chicken or tofu with a rainbow salad or a bowl of vegetable-rich pasta. These options provide key proteins and a cornucopia of vitamins and minerals.

Evening Snack – Keep Metabolism Active: Opt for Greek yogurt topped with probiotic-rich fermented foods like kimchi or a handful of nuts and seeds. This snack aids digestion while providing a dose of essential minerals and probiotics.

Dinner – Wrap Up Right: Round off the day with a plate of grilled fish and steamed vegetables or a wholesome chickpea curry with brown rice. These meals deliver immune-strengthening nutrients in a delicious, comforting finale.

With this planning, remember that variety is key—not only to keep your diet exciting but also to ensure you're getting a wide range of nutrients.

7.3. Modifying Your Diet: Dietary Restriction Considerations

Nutrition is personal, and dietary restrictions—whether due to allergies, intolerances, or dietary preferences—should always be considered. For example, vegetarians and vegans can replace animal proteins with plant-based options like lentils, beans, and tofu while those who are gluten intolerant can opt for gluten-free grains such as quinoa, rice, and amaranth.

7.4. Staying Hydrated

Don't forget the importance of hydration. Water plays a crucial role in carrying nutrients to cells and flushing out toxins. Aim for at least eight glasses a day.

7.5. Shifting Towards A Healthy Lifestyle

Diet is only one piece of the immunity puzzle. Adequate sleep, regular exercise, stress management, and refraining from harmful habits like smoking and excessive drinking are all integral to building a strong immune system.

Planning meals focused on immune-boosting nutrients is a fantastic strategy to build a robust defense system. Remember, the journey to an immune-rich lifestyle isn't a destination but a continuous process. So, take the plunge, experiment with food, and nourish your body the right way!

Chapter 8. Breaking Down the Science: How Fitness and Nutrition Strengthen Immunity

Immunity is our body's biological defense system designed to shield us from disease-causing organisms and potentially damaging foreign bodies. Essentially, it is our body's personal health guard, tirelessly working round the clock to ensure we stay protected from infections, viruses, and diseases. Nutrition and fitness play an integral role in fortifying this guard, empowering each individual to control their health destiny effectively.

8.1. The Science Of Immunity

In simple terms, our immune system is a complex network of cells, tissues, and organs working harmoniously to keep our body protected. It can be broadly divided into two components: innate and adaptive immunity. Innate immunity serves as our first line of defense, reacting quickly to any perceived threats. Conversely, adaptive immunity takes time to respond; however, it develops a memory of previous attacks, allowing a more rapid and efficient defense upon reinfection.

Maintaining an optimal immune response requires regular training and nourishment – something fitness and nutrition can greatly play into. Our thymus, bone marrow, and lymphatic system generate and train immune cells. Their optimal functioning can actually be facilitated through regular exercise and a balanced diet, enabling a potent defense mechanism against pathogens.

8.2. The Role Of Fitness In Immunity

Physical activity has long been associated with a broad range of health benefits, and enhancing immunity is one of them. Exercise furthers the effective circulation of immune cells, helping them to reach all areas of the body more promptly and efficiently. This heightened immune cell mobility gives your body an edge, as it allows for a faster response to possible threats.

Moreover, regular physical activity can help reduce inflammation, which has a crucial part in many autoimmune diseases. Studies have shown that moderate-intensity exercise can lead to a temporary rise in anti-inflammatory responses.

Physical fitness also aids in stress management, which is crucial to maintaining a healthy immune system. Being in a chronic state of stress can overwork the immune system, leaving it less capable of effectively responding to microbes and infections. Exercise helps reduce these stress levels, thus aiding in balance and optimum functioning of our immune system.

8.3. Nutrient-rich Diet For A Robust Immunity

While physical activity tones our immunity, a premium fuel in the form of nutrition-dense foods ensures it runs smoothly. Certain nutrients have been scientifically proven to be essential for the proper functioning of our immune system. Vitamins A, C, D, and E, along with minerals like selenium, zinc, iron, and proteins, play key roles in maintaining and enhancing our immunity.

Let's discuss those in detail:

- **Vitamin A**: This vitamin aids in the growth of immune cells and produces an antibody response. Foods rich in Vitamin A include sweet potatoes, spinach, and carrots.

- **Vitamin C**: Acts as an antioxidant and can speed up the recovery process. Daily intake can be sourced from fruits like oranges, kiwi, and vegetables like bell peppers.

- **Vitamin D**: Integral to immune response activation and can be obtained through sun exposure and foods like fatty fish, cheese, and egg yolks.

- **Vitamin E**: An antioxidant that helps protect immune cells. Can be found in nuts and seeds.

- **Zinc**: Essential for the development of immune cells and can be obtained through meat, shellfish, and legumes.

- **Selenium**: Helps lower oxidative stress, enhancing immunity. This nutrient can be sourced from seafood, nuts, and seeds.

- **Iron**: Assists in the growth of immune cells and antibodies. It's chiefly found in poultry, meat, fish, and leafy greens.

- **Protein**: Essential for the formation of antibodies, obtained through both plant (nuts, legumes) and animal sources (meat, dairy, eggs).

Ensuring a balanced and diverse diet can help cater to these nutrient needs, fortifying our immune system from within.

8.4. Fostering Healthy Habits: Fitness and Nutrition Routine

Now that we understand how fitness and nutrition bolster our immune health, we need to translate this knowledge into actionable steps and foster healthy habits. The key to successful integration is a gradual shift towards more nutritious meals and regular physical activity. Starting small, like including a portion of fruits and vegetables at each meal or adopting a 15-minute daily walk, can go a long way as these small steps eventually amalgamate into a transformative lifestyle shift.

By fusing science-backed advice with practical lifestyle changes, we can gear our body's defense mechanism to function at its best, fortifying our immunity, and enhancing our overall health and wellbeing. Remember, every step counts towards the healthier, fitter version of yourself you aspire to be. Embrace the journey!

However, it's crucial to acknowledge that each body is unique, and therefore, health strategies are not 'one-size-fits-all.' Always consider individual health needs, personal preferences, and consult a healthcare provider before significantly changing your diet or starting an exercise routine.

In the end, total wellness is about more than just staving off illness. It's about thriving, living life with vitality - and fitness and nutrition are both paramount to that journey. Your body is capable of incredible things. Feed it well, keep it moving, and watch the magic happen as you pave the way towards an improved immune function and a revitalized life.

Chapter 9. Mindfulness and Meditation: Secret Weapons for a Stronger Immunity

As we dive into the fascinating world of mindfulness and meditation, it's crucial to lay the groundwork with a clear understanding of what these concepts involve. Mindfulness, born from Buddhist traditions, refers to the state of being fully present, aware of where we are and what we are doing. It is about not getting overly reactive or overwhelmed by what's going on around us. More specifically, Mindfulness-Based Stress Reduction (MBSR), pioneered by Dr. Jon Kabat-Zinn, has been widely recognized for its instrumental role in integrating mindfulness into modern medicine.

Meditation, often intertwined with mindfulness, is a broad term that encompasses various techniques designed to promote relaxation, build internal energy, and develop love, patience, empathy, and forgiveness, among others. Though the techniques may vary, the intended results are generally the same: a mind that is quiet, concentrated, and lucid.

9.1. Syncing Mind and Body for Enhanced Immunity

Let's examine the intricate connections between mindfulness, meditation, and the immune system's functioning. Our immune system, a complex network of cells, organs, and chemicals, acts as our body's defense against pathogens, viruses, and diseases. When our immune system is not at its best, we are more susceptible to illness.

There is a strong established link between our mental state and our physical health. Chronic stress, anxiety, and depression can wreak havoc on our immune system, reducing its capacity to fight off illnesses. This is where mindfulness and meditation come into play. By quieting the mind, reducing stress, and promoting mental health, these practices indirectly enhance our body's resilience against diseases.

Several scientific studies have spotlighted the beneficial impacts of mindfulness and meditation on the immune system. A 2003 study by Davidson et al. noted that participants who underwent eight weeks of mindfulness meditation training showed significant increases in left-sided anterior activation, a brain pattern associated with positive affect, and immune function.

9.2. Your Guide to Mindfulness and Meditation

Now that we've established the foundations of mindfulness and meditation and their relation to the immune system, let's go on a journey to understand how to integrate these practices into your everyday life.

For beginners, it can be helpful to start with short, daily meditation sessions. Find a quiet and comfortable place where you can sit down, relax, and focus. The beauty of mindfulness and meditation lies in their universality – you don't need any special equipment or a specific setting. All it requires is your presence, commitment, and patience.

Practicing mindful breathing (or conscious breathing) is one of the easiest ways to bring mindfulness into your life. It's a simple yet powerful method, and it goes as follow:

- Find a comfortable sitting or lying position.

- Close your eyes and take a deep breath in, noticing the sensation of your lungs filling with air, your chest rising.

- Exhale slowly. Stay focused on your breath's rhythm and feel your body relax with each outgoing breath.

- If your mind begins to wander, gently guide it back to your breath without judgment.

- Continue this practice for 5-10 minutes every day, gradually increasing the duration as you become more comfortable with the practice.

9.3. Combine Mindfulness with Exercise

Physical exercises like yoga, tai chi, or qigong incorporate mindfulness principles, and they offer health benefits beyond regular exercise. Harmonizing breath and movement, these disciplines enhance body awareness and promote improved physical and mental health. They're also fun to do!

Yoga, an ancient practice that originates from India, involves a series of physical postures (or asanas) combined with breath control and meditation. Regular yoga practice has been shown to help lower blood pressure, improve heart function, and bolster the immune system.

Tai chi and qigong, both Chinese martial arts forms, also fuse slow, deliberate movements, meditation, and regulated breath. Practitioners highlight their benefits in reducing stress, improving mood, and enhancing immune function. These routines can be a perfect addition to your morning or evening rituals.

9.4. The Practice of Mindful Eating

We are what we eat—an age-old adage that holds a lot of truth. Good nutrition is a key propeller in boosting our immune system and keeping us well. Mindful eating is a practice that involves being fully present when eating, savoring every bite, and consciously choosing the foods that nourish us both physically and mentally.

To adopt mindful eating, start with these small steps:

- Chew slowly and focus on the flavors, textures, and aromas of your food.

- Acknowledge your hunger and fullness cues and use them to decide when to start and stop eating.

- Appreciate your food and consider its journey from source to plate.

- Minimize distractions (like your phone or TV) while eating.

- Make healthy food choices; opt for fruits, vegetables, lean proteins, and whole-grain foods that can strengthen your immune system.

In conclusion, the secret weapons to a stronger immune system could very well be within us. By embracing mindfulness and meditation, we can foster a calming environment within our bodies that promotes physical wellness, resistance to diseases, and overall better health. While the world outside can get chaotic, let's invest in cultivating the tranquility within, for the health benefits are profound and far-reaching. Welcome to a revitalized life!

Chapter 10. Supplements and Vitamins: A Comprehensive Guide for Extra Support

In the quest for optimum health and robust immunity, it is important to understand the role that supplements and vitamins play in complementing our dietary needs. Supplements cannot substitute a nutrient-rich, balanced diet; however, they can provide additional support when nutrient demands increase or when consuming a specific nutrient becomes challenging.

10.1. Understanding the Basics

The first step in comprehensively analyzing supplements and vitamins is understanding what they are and how they function. Simply put, dietary supplements are products containing one or more dietary ingredients, like vitamins, minerals, amino acids, or herbs—and are intended to supplement our diet. They come in various forms such as tablets, capsules, softgels, gelcaps, powders, or liquids.

Vitamins are complex, organic compounds essential for normal growth, metabolism, and overall wellbeing. They're divided into two groups: water-soluble vitamins (B-complex vitamins and vitamin C), which are not stored in the body and must be replenished daily, and fat-soluble vitamins (vitamins A, D, E, and K), which are stored in the fat cells of the body and liver.

10.2. Role of Vitamins in Immune Function

Each vitamin uniquely contributes to immune function. Vitamins A, C, D, E, and B6, for instance, play an integral role.

Vitamin A, also known as retinol, supports the health of the skin and tissue lining the gut, lungs, and other parts of the body, providing a first line of defense against infections.

Vitamin C, also recognized as ascorbic acid, acts as an antioxidant and plays a crucial part in supporting cellular functions of the immune system. It contributes to the skin's defense system, stimulates the production of white blood cells, and can also enhance their functioning.

Vitamin D is known to enhance the innate immune response and modulate the adaptive immune response, reducing the risk of infection. It can be synthesized by the human body when exposed to sunlight, making it a unique vitamin.

Vitamin E is a potent antioxidant that helps combat oxidative stress, which can negatively impact immune health if left unregulated.

Vitamin B6 is critical for supporting biochemical reactions in the immune system, and deficiency can influence immune response.

10.3. Reasoning Behind Supplements

Even though the human body can produce few vitamins itself, most vitamins must be procured from food or dietary supplements because the body either doesn't produce enough or doesn't produce them at all. Incorporating supplements can contribute to maintaining optimal vitamin levels, particularly for vitamins that are not sufficiently obtained from food sources.

10.4. Evaluating Your Supplement Needs

Before beginning a supplement regimen, it's essential to evaluate your individual needs, which can be influenced by your eating habits, age, lifestyle, and health conditions.

Pregnant women, for example, require a higher intake of nutrients like folic acid, iron, and calcium. Adults over 50 might need additional B12, which can be difficult to absorb from food sources. Vegetarians and vegans might benefit from iron, zinc, iodine, calcium, and vitamins D and B12 supplements, as these nutrients are predominantly found in animal products. People with limited sun exposure may require vitamin D supplements.

10.5. Selecting the Right Products

With countless supplements available, choosing the right one can seem daunting. Start by checking for third-party testing from groups like NSF, USP, or ConsumerLab, ensuring the product meets quality measures for safety and efficacy.

Consider the dosage too; the Recommended Dietary Allowance (RDA) for each nutrient serves as a valuable guide. Do not exceed the Upper Intake Level (UL) - the maximum amount unlikely to cause adverse health effects.

10.6. Potential Risks and Consult Your Healthcare Provider

Supplements should be used wisely. Excessive dosage of certain supplements, such as vitamin A or iron, can cause serious health problems. Fat-soluble vitamins, if consumed excessively, can accumulate in the body and lead to toxicity. Always consult a healthcare provider before starting any supplement regimen.

In conclusion, understanding the role and source of each vitamin, along with your unique dietary needs, will help you make informed decisions about supplementation. Supplements and vitamins represent an important piece of the puzzle to holistic health and enhanced immunity, not as replacements but as reinforcements to a balanced diet and other healthy lifestyle practices.

Chapter 11. Your Immunity Transformation: A 30-Day Action Plan

We all have a natural guard that protects us from germs and viruses—a system that keeps us healthy, vibrant and brimming with energy—the immune system. This chapter details a comprehensive 30-day action plan that will take your immunity from ordinary to extraordinary, replenishing your body and endowing you with a fortified defense mechanism. Based on scientifically backed fitness exercises and nutritional habits, this systematic regimen is designed to be easy-to-follow and effectively transforms your immunity landscape. Let's start this journey to a stronger version of yourself.

11.1. Understand the Role of Nutrients in Boosting Immunity

Nutrition plays a pivotal role in our overall health and significantly influences our immune functions. Over the next 30 days, it's vital to understand the importance of tailored meals and specific nutrients that are key in boosting our immunity.

Micro nutrients such as vitamins A, B6, C, and E, along with minerals like zinc, selenium, and iron are famed superstars in the realm of immunity. These, along with other nutrients such as omega-3 fatty acids, polyphenols, and dietary fiber, are known to support and enhance the immune response. A combination of a rich nutrient-based diet can enhance your immune defense and provide optimal health benefits.

11.2. Follow a 4-Week Immune-Boosting Meal Plan

Incorporating an immunity-rich diet doesn't have to be complicated. Use the following 4-week meal plan as a guide. It includes foods loaded with immunity-boosting nutrients that you can easily add to your daily meals.

1. Week 1: Begin with a focus on Vitamin C, which has been found to boost immunity by stimulating the production of white blood cells. Foods high in Vitamin C include citrus fruits, tomatoes, strawberries, and red bell peppers.

2. Week 2: Switch your focus to Vitamin A, notably found in plant-based foods like sweet potatoes, pumpkins, and dark leafy green vegetables. Vitamin A plays a vital role in maintaining the health of your natural barriers, such as skin, which helps prevent bacteria from entering the body.

3. Week 3: Now turn your attention to foods rich in Zinc. These include legumes, nuts, and seeds—particularly pumpkin seeds. Zinc is crucial to the effective functioning of the immune system as it is required for the production of white blood cells.

4. Week 4: Lastly, focus on maintaining a consistent diet replete with all these nutrients. Ensure your days are packed with a variety of fruits, vegetables, legumes, nuts, and seeds.

Remember, hydration is a critical part of the process, so drink plenty of water alongside your meals.

11.3. The Power of Fitness in Immunity Enhancement

Regular exercise is a cornerstone of a healthier lifestyle and a stronger immune system. Keeping such notions at the crux, our 30-

day fitness regimen focuses on combining cardio, strength training, flexibility exercises, and relaxation techniques to enhance your immune function.

1. Week 1: Engage in moderate-intensity cardio exercises such as brisk walking, cycling, or swimming for 30 minutes a day, five days a week. Cardio exercises increase your breathing rate, which may help your immune system perform more effectively.

2. Week 2: Introduce one to two days of strength training. Exercises such as weightlifting or bodyweight routines help build muscle mass and strengthen the body, which supports a healthy immune system.

3. Week 3: Advanced level cardio. Take your cardio routine up a notch by increasing the intensity or duration of your exercises. You can also try adding interval training to your routine.

4. Week 4: Blend in flexibility stretches and relaxation exercises such as yoga and meditation. This synergic amalgamation benefits your immune system by reducing stress hormones in the body. Remember, stress can hinder the functioning of your immune system, keeping it in check is essential.

11.4. Rest To Revitalize

It is during sleep that our body rebuilds, repairs itself, and maintains a strong immune system. Not getting enough rest may decrease the production of essential immune cells and can leave you more prone to infections. Make sleep a priority, aim for 7-9 hours each night.

11.5. Tune Into Better Lifestyle Choices

Besides diet and exercise, lifestyle habits play an important role in optimizing our immunity. Reducing stress levels, abstaining from smoking, limiting alcohol intake, and ensuring proper hygiene practices can significantly boost your immune system health.

Over these 30 days, make a conscious effort to replace one bad habit with one good one—one step at a time. Remember, small changes contribute to big differences in the long run.

11.6. Search for Support

If you find yourself struggling to maintain the 30-day plan, recruit a friend or family member to join you. A support system can help you stay motivated and transform your journey into a fun and engaging experience.

By following this 30-day action plan, you are laying the groundwork for a stronger immune system, better health, and an enriched life. Start today; your journey toward superior immunity and incredible health awaits you! Remember, the key to your health lies within you, tap into it and unlock a life full of vigor and vital force.